"I have known Angelique for over 30 years, and when she was diagnosed with breast cancer, I went on the journey with her through her blog. I would have never guessed, that three years later, I would be going through that same journey. The first person I reached out to after my diagnoses was her. She was basically my "cancer coach". She prepared me for every step of the way, and I am still so grateful to her! I could not have been more prepared for each hurdle that I had to cross."

— Cathy Williamson, www.the-middlepage.com,
Cancer Survivor

"You have your own "Angelique wisdom file" on my computer where I save all your emails for future reference and support. I love you sharing your story and the idea of finding a way to let other people be as lucky as I am to be living it step by step with you. I can't tell you how comforting it is. Thanks for being on this journey with me. I feel you with me every step of the way and am so grateful for that and your beacon of light."

— Barb Burg Schieffelin, VP,
Global Head of Communications Thomson Reuters

"Being diagnosed with cancer was devastating beyond any-thing I could imagine. I reached out to Angelique because I knew she had been through it. She was compassionate yet tough. She answered my questions and provided support. In answering my questions she shared her journey and in sup-porting me she shared what worked best for her and others she knew. Angelique helped me create balance in my life, when I was thrown off kilter, through her stories and advice."

— Theresa Chutuk, Cancer Survivor

Chemo
Cupcakes
AND
Carpools

HOW TO GO THROUGH CHEMO
WITH YOUR FAMILY, YOUR MARRIAGE,
AND YOUR SANITY INTACT

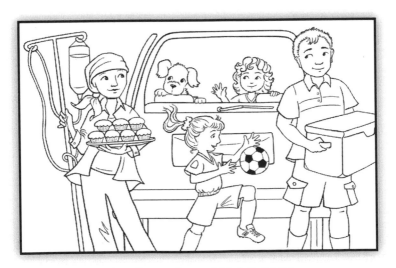

ANGELIQUE L'AMOUR

Chemo, Cupcakes And Carpools

How to go through chemo with your family,
your marriage and your sanity intact.

Angelique L'Amour
Angelique L'Amour Pitney, Pub

Published by Angelique L'Amour Pitney Publishing,
Los Angeles County, CA

Editor: Lisbeth Tanz, lisbethtanz.com

Cover illustration and design: Denise Clemmensen, deniseclemmensen.com

Interior design: DavisCreative.com

ISBN: 978-0-9975444-1-1

ATTENTION CORPORATIONS, UNIVERSITIES, COLLEGES AND PROFESSIONAL ORGANIZATIONS: Quantity discounts are available on bulk purchases of this book for educational and gift purposes or as premiums for increasing magazine subscriptions or renewals. Special books or book excerpts can also be created to fit specific needs. For information, please contact Angelique L'Amour Pitney at Angelique@angeliquelamour.com)

For Barb—
who asked for this first

Medical Disclaimer

The medical information on this in this book is provided as an information resource only, and is not to be used or relied on for any diagnostic or treatment purposes. This information is not intended to be patient education, does not create any patient-physician relationship, and should not be used as a substitute for professional diagnosis and treatment.

Please consult your health care provider before making any healthcare decisions or for guidance about a specific medical condition. The author, Angelique L'Amour Pitney, AKA Angelique L'Amour, expressly disclaims responsibility, and shall have no liability, for any damages, loss, injury, or liability whatsoever suffered as a result of your reliance on the information contained in this book. Angelique L'Amour Pitney does not endorse specifically any test, treatment, or procedure mentioned in this book, it is meant to be informative only.

By reading this book you agree to the foregoing terms and conditions, which may from time to time be changed or supplemented by the author. If you do not agree to the foregoing terms and conditions, you should not read this book.

Acknowledgments

Thank you to my husband, Christopher Pitney and our daughters, Kate and Sarah for standing by me, supporting me, and reminding me to laugh.

Thank you to my MHS sisters for encouraging me and for helping with the title—it was a group effort all around.

Thank you to Cathy Williamson and Teresa Chutuk for being my first readers.

Thank you to Lisbeth Tanz—for the first eyes on this and her help and encouragement.

Thank you to Cathy Davis for the beautiful design.

Thank you to Karen Garcia for keeping my i's and t's in their proper positions.

Table of Contents

Introduction 1

1: I have cancer; how do I tell my kids? 2

2: What kind of help will I need? 6

3: What should I do before treatment begins? 10

4: What can spouses, family members, and friends do? 14

5: What is a PORT? 18

6: What will the treatment and after affects be like? 22

7: How can I look good while going through treatment? . . . 28

8: Side Effects 34

9: How do I deal with sick friends and relatives
   (not to mention perfect strangers)? 40

10: What do I eat? Will I eat? 44

11: How do I find faith, friends, and moments to myself? . . 48

12: Should I troll the Internet
    – AKA – The Court of Public Opinion? 50

13: Will I feel like exercising? 54

14: How do I volunteer at school? 58

15: Why did I start burning the pancakes? 62

16: How did I make decisions? 66

Questions and Helpful Hints in a Nut Shell;
AKA Troubleshooting Guide 71

Glossary 75

Helpful Things 77

About the Author 79

About the Cover Artist 81

Introduction

I am a mom. I am not a doctor. This is not medical advice; it is practical advice. Over the last six years, I have been asked many times for advice on surviving time in the cancer trenches. The questions were sometimes about medical things, but more often, they were about how to handle lives in the midst of cancer treatment. How do I tell my kids? What kind of help will I need? How will I feel? How do I deal with my hair? Each time I would write an email outlining all the helpful hints I used and send it off. As time went by, I kept that email and improved upon it and would send virtually the same one.

Just as I was ending my chemo, a dear friend was beginning her journey. She kept saying to me, "You need to write the 'Girlfriend's Guide to Chemo' book." Like the ones written by Vicky Iovine, whose books we devoured as pregnant women and then as new moms. As I began writing, I realized there were two books I wanted to write. One book would be about my journey and experiences; the other, a helpful hints type of book for moms and dads dealing with a cancer diagnosis while taking care of their families.

What follows is mom advice. Everything I say needs to be run by your doctors. EVERY. SINGLE. THING. This book will give you one way to navigate your journey. You can read how I did it, and see what works for you. I sincerely hope this helps you in your journey.

I have cancer;
how do I
tell my kids?

My girls were ages 7 and 11 when I was diagnosed. I called a friend who was a psychiatrist and asked him this very question. His answer caught me off guard.

"Don't tell them," he advised. Not tell my kids?

I couldn't imagine anything that would add more pressure to my life than trying to hide this from them. We were— and are—very close. Not telling them would have been impossible.

After another meeting with my doctor, I decided I was having a double mastectomy. As a stay-at-home mom, I was about to disappear for a week, and it wasn't to take a vacation. I rarely traveled without them, so I knew it was only a matter of time before I had to tell them.

My oldest had a friend whose mom had breast cancer. In addition, this mom was BRCA positive, so my daughter knew a little more about breast cancer than the average 11-year-old did. I didn't have much time to decide how to tell her as she has always been in tune with me; plus, she heard me making an appointment on the phone.

She straight up asked, "Do you have cancer?"

I replied, "Yes, and I have to have surgery. I have breast cancer."

We then went for a fast walk around the neighborhood. I wanted to speak to her without her little sister so she could ask me anything without being overheard. She asked all her questions, and I answered them one by one. I didn't say that I would be fine. I told her the plan was that I would be fine, and that I would be in the hospital and then at her grandmother's house for about a week. She asked if I would lose my hair. I said I didn't know yet. She is a bright and sophisticated kid, so I answered her straight but didn't elaborate on anything I didn't know for sure. She made it easy because she asked. Her sister was different.

My youngest was seven and I kept it simple.

"I have something called cancer, and I have to have surgery to take it out. Some people think cancer is a scary word and get worried. I don't think it is a scary word. I will be gone for a week or so in the hospital and at my mom's. We can talk on the phone."

I also had to tell her that when I came home, we couldn't bear hug for a bit as I would be healing and sore, but she could hug me gently as much as she wanted. She didn't have specific questions. She just wanted me to read to her, which was something completely normal.

When they asked if I would be okay, I said, "That's the plan." When they asked if I would die, I said, "The plan is that I will live until I am old and a grandma or great grandma." No drama just straight talk, and I didn't dwell on the word choice. I was aware that I wasn't promising to be there forever, so I just lightly used the words, "The plan is ..."

You have to decide what to tell your kids based on their age and experience. Let them lead with their questions and don't embellish.

- Keep it simple.

- Answer the questions that are asked.

- Don't make promises until you know you can make them come true.

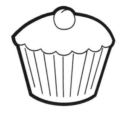

What kind of help
will I need?

The short answer is ... all the help you can get. If your chemo is like mine, which was every 21 days, you will feel pretty lousy for the first five days and then start to feel better.

A quick note: in this book I will refer to the day of chemo as day one and count the days to the next chemo from that point onward.

On days one and two, you will need the most help from someone else. Then on day three and four I was tired and achy. I could have driven my kids the short distance to and from school the day after chemo; but by days three and four, I was grateful that I didn't have to. By day five, I was feeling better. Driving and other activities were easier. I felt what I called "chemo fine."

"Chemo fine" is a state where you feel fine to do some normal things, but you tire easily, and by 7:00 p.m., you are done. I would push through the homework, dinner, bath, and bed routine. Most nights, however, the kids went to bed at 8:00 p.m.—an hour after me! Then on day 21 it all started again.

Having someone to help with the housekeeping is really, really nice. In fact, I would say it is a great present if someone wants to give you something. You need your rest as you are healing, plus you don't feel great. I found I could still cook. I spent some of my downtime in bed watching cooking shows and planning meals. Yes, I was nauseous, but it didn't bother me to watch those shows! I had enough energy that I could have cleaned my house after the chemo week was over, but I was lucky enough to have help.

Carpools are a great idea. You can return the favor the next week. Knowing your kids are getting where they need to go frees your brain from worry, and not driving gives you more time to rest and be ready for after school responsibilities. One of my goals was to keep their lives as normal and as consistent as possible. Other parents helped a great deal keeping the kids able to go to the events and parties without having to miss anything because I didn't feel up to it.

Both my girls were playing soccer that year, and I relied on the parents from my older daughter's team. Often, the parents would send their kids over to play with my oldest, which meant I could rest or spend time with my youngest. These same parents always picked their kids up on time and understood the rule about healthy kids only at my house. It was a win-win for everyone! My oldest was on a club team so there were nights when she stayed at a teammate's house so I could sleep in a bit. I still went to her games, but I didn't always have to do the early wakeup, breakfast, pack snacks thing.

My younger daughter also had play dates, but mostly ones that took place outside since seven-year-olds still tend to get sick a lot. It was important for me to avoid getting sick so I could do my chemo treatments on time.

It may be hard at first to accept help, but it is vitally important you accept what is offered and ask for what you really need.

- Say yes to people who offer to help. You may not need them, but it is better to have help lined up.

- Get rides for chemo day for you and chemo day plus two more for your kids.

- Let other parents know you won't need them to drive every day and that you will return the favor the next week.

- Housekeeping help is terrific, at least for chemo week.

What should
I do before
treatment begins?

The Before Treatment Begins Checklist:

1. Driving the kids:

Get rides for the kids together, at least for the chemo week.

2. Dealing with meals:

You will be able to cook, but the first two to three days it is nice not to have to make dinner. The end of the day was always a push until 7:00 p.m. when I could disappear to my bedroom, take some medicine, and fall asleep. The tiredness did seem to stay with me through the month, but it was not as bad once I was through the first five days. Honestly, it was easier for my husband or friends to bring take out than for anyone to cook, and it was only a matter of a day or two.

3. Taking care of other medical business:

See your dentist before you start chemo, because your doctor won't want you getting your teeth cleaned or having a filling while going through chemo.

Ask your oncologist if you need shots (flu, pneumonia, shingles, etc.), before beginning treatment. I was going through chemo during a particularly bad flu season.

4. Automating your bills:

I put everything I could on auto pay using my credit cards because I didn't trust the process of letting my creditors withdraw money from my bank account directly. I still don't. Besides, I earned frequent flyer mileage! I did set up online bill paying through my bank in case I chose to pay a bill that way. It did make paying bills easier for me—and it will for you, too Trust me. You won't feel like paying bills, so make it easy to get that chore done.

5. Spiffing yourself up:

Get a manicure and pedicure from a clean place. You likely won't have another one for a while as you won't want to risk getting an infection from a mani/pedi or sick from the people in the salon. Remember that your immune system is about to be taxed, and you will have to be more careful than you usually would. It's probably best to stay with clear polish for now, which means getting rid of the gels and acrylics. It is possible your nails will be affected by the chemo treatment. You want to be able to see this and care for anything that comes up.

Get your hair done even if you will be losing it during treatments. A nice haircut or style will help you feel better before that happens. Some people cut their hair short in advance. I didn't, but I did color it. I didn't want my gray to show before it fell out! After it starts to grow back, you should have a trim earlier than you would think. Just cleaning up the edges of your inch long (or shorter) hair will make it all look better. I was surprised at the boost it gave me when my hairdresser trimmed my hair after cutting the girls. My hair must have been less than one-half inch long, but that trim made it look better, which made me feel better.

6. Protecting yourself:

Buy surgical masks for when you have to be in a crowd (school play, church). You don't have to be stuck with boring white ones as there are many fashionable and colorful ones you can purchase online.

Buy hand sanitizer for your house, car, kitchen, bedside table, purse, backpacks, and lunchboxes.

7. Organizing your chemo entertainment:

I did a variety of things while getting treatment –

- Bought a laptop and started a blog
- Started a new knitting project
- Found a new book and a series of books to read
- Completed my Christmas shopping online (using my new laptop)
- Emailed friends. This is a great time to see who might want to come with you the next time. The time in the chemo chair is fairly boring, which is a good thing.

What can spouses,
family members,
and friends do?

Your spouse, friends, and family members will want to know how to help.

You may need and want a companion to go with you to tests and appointments. At some point, you can stop hearing what is being said to you. It is also good to have someone with you to listen and ask questions. My friend took her 25-year-old daughter. I went alone to most things as our kids were little, and I needed my husband to be with them. He came to chemo, and he came to the first doctor's appointment or two. I did the scans by myself. I thought I could handle it—that is until I experienced delays in my final implant surgery resulting from a bout of pneumonia and a scary lung pet scan. Suddenly, my doctor started to sound like the adults in a Peanuts cartoon, "Mua Mua Mua." It was truly weird and can happen at any point in this journey. When it happened to me, I insisted that my husband come with me to my next appointment.

Some friends may offer to grocery shop for you or pick up take out. A few non-profits offer house cleaning for women in treatment.

My greatest challenge after my initial surgery was dog grooming. Don't laugh! I have a standard Labradoodle, and he is big. After my initial surgery, it took me four separate times to groom his entire body. I also needed help running the kids around (that's where carpooling is invaluable). It's also helpful to have someone around while the kids are home if your spouse is gone. This allows you to go to bed if you need to and know the kids are looked after and fed.

My mom offered to keep a treatment bill log and insurance log. You will have more bills and EOBs than you can imagine, and having someone manage the paperwork is a huge help. I would also ask for a ride to and from events at school when my spouse couldn't take me and driving myself wasn't an option.

Remember spouses want to DO something, so help them by asking for what you need. Your family and friends will feel helpless, so just say yes when people offer. This is perhaps the hardest thing but you will need help sometimes, so you might as well say yes. You can always say, "Yes, I will need help, but I don't know how yet."

One neighbor simply called and said, "I am going to Whole Foods. What would you like?"

I answered, "A roasted chicken." My other neighbor simply dropped off a bag of salad and some bread one day.

- Say "Yes"!
- Ask for help!

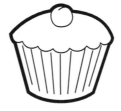

What is
a PORT?

When your doctor suggests you get a port, just say, "Thank you," and do it.

Ports, also known as a port-a-cath, are a great gift. I have strong veins, and I wanted to keep them that way. I was only 45 when I was diagnosed, so getting a port was important. I didn't want to have trouble with my veins ever, and so I needed to take this step. A small valve is placed under the skin in the chest or arm with a catheter attached. This port essentially provides a line into your bloodstream 24/7 to accept medications, such as chemo or antibiotics, or to give blood for blood tests. Ports require a large vein, which is why they are typically located in the upper arm or chest area. Once you have a port placed you will only have to have it accessed through the skin rather than always searching for a vein to use.

It sounds easy, but I was freaked about it. Much more so than about the mastectomy! Then I met this delicate, beautiful, 6-year-old girl with cystic fibrosis. SHE had had a port placed four times. When she spoke to me and told me about how she had a port here and here and here and here, I no longer worried about myself. She was strong enough for me to feel like a fool for worrying.

Some doctors place these under general anesthesia and some under local. Mine was a local, and the doctor and nurses were great about it. One nurse even held my hand while the procedure was taking place.

Before your chemo treatment, you will be given numbing cream to apply before you get to the infusion center. Put it on like you're frosting a cupcake! This is not face cream. Put a glob on, and cover it with a bandage that is sticky all the way around it. You will feel pressure but no pain when they access your port during chemo.

- Say yes to the port.

- Frost a cupcake with the Lidocaine cream!

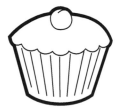

What will the
treatment and
after affects be like?

One of the best pieces of advice I can give you is to write things down. EVERYTHING. Record how you feel after chemo the first time, what medicine you took for side effects, and how you managed the first week. This is your roadmap forward. Writing this information down is great because it allows us to plan. A certain amount of lousy is to be expected, but it doesn't happen every day of those 21. At first, I wrote on my calendar how I felt each day, what I took and if it worked, and then blogged about it at Mystoryrightnow.blogspot.com. If you go back to the archives for 2009-2010, you will see my notes. Writing things down will also help you keep track of your medication schedule.

Since I wrote how I felt, what I took, how it helped or didn't, 21 days later I could do the same things or try different ones. People will say, "It's cumulative," and give you a knowing look with a nod of the head. Truthfully, unless they have gone through it, they don't know. I tried to ignore unhelpful attitudes and keep myself surrounded by positive people to help me stay positive. For me, the medicine effects didn't get harder as I went along; but I did become less patient with my life coming to a full stop every 21 days while I recovered from yet another treatment. I also felt a big change when I stopped taking oral steroids, as they helped me get back on my feet. I did have a friend who felt the effects were cumulative. She was on entirely different medicine from me, and she did radiation as well. Everyone's reaction is different. That is why you need to write it down; it will help you plan your life in the middle of all of it.

Everyone's cocktail of chemo is different as well, so don't compare; but since I know you are curious, I will tell you. I did six treatments of Taxotere and Carboplatin with Herceptin and 12 of Herceptin alone. I was in the chemo chair for a year, but only the first six treatments were the really tough ones. For the following 12 treatments, I drove myself. I made sure to drink a lot of water and a bottle of Gatorade on treatment day because my side effect from Herceptin was dehydration.

My first chemo treatment was anticlimactic. I grew up in the 1970s and 80s. All the movies from that era made chemo look dramatic—a lot of throwing up and passing out dramatic. Back then it probably was like that. Now there are great side effect drugs and nutritional help.

When I arrived for my chemo, they checked my blood and then, after a bit, started my drip. Three bags of clear chemo fluid and about five hours later, I was done. I felt woozy from the Benadryl they put in my drip. I asked them to do that again each time as it made sitting in the chair easier, like a glass of wine or a tranquilizer. I also sucked on ice cubes the first time in hopes that the mouth sores wouldn't be too bad. From then on, I just bought an iced organic mint lemonade iced tea with extra ice and kept my mouth cold. I also iced my fingers and toes as one of the side effects of my drugs was the possibility of losing my finger-nails and toenails.

Getting chemo is not exciting. In fact, most days were boring. During all my treatments, I had a book, magazines, and my laptop (my chemo buddy in electronic form). I had my mom and husband to keep me company.

During all my chemo treatments, I also wrote both my blog and emails. I graded papers. I did my Christmas shopping and wrote Christmas cards. I was teaching both creative writing and literature to sixth graders, and I had some work to do. The kids were aware of what was going on. I taught in the classroom before I started chemo. After it started, I taught via Skype until chemo was over.

After my first treatment, I felt somewhat disconnected—high almost. That feeling was due to the massive amount of Benadryl and other drugs in my system. My mom drove me to her house where I could rest undisturbed.

Expect the unexpected. A distressing side effect I experienced at dinner that first night was a completely dry throat and mouth. I wasn't sure what caused this; it could have been the chemo, but it could have been the Benadryl, too. This side effect arrived after each chemo and lasted less than a day. The problem was easily handled by taking a sip of water with every bite of food, but I had to concentrate so I didn't choke.

The next day, I went back for the hydration that my center offered. I also got a Neulasta shot to boost my immune system. I was told to take Claritin the day of the shot to help with the bone pain which can be a result of the shot.,

A month later, I was taking Claritin for my allergies, which seemed worse since I had lost my nose hair (yes, it really falls out from all parts of your body). There was quite a difference between taking the Claritin the day before my shot and the day of the shot. It worked better for me to take it the day before to prevent the bone pain, but ASK YOUR DOCTOR!

One of the drugs I was on led to weakened fingernails and toenails. Since my nails weren't strong to begin with, I needed to do what I could to keep them. To reduce the chance I would lose them, I iced my fingers and toes. Icing actually helps to keep nails from falling off. It was uncomfortable, but worth it.

- Write it down: appointments, what drugs you have taken, and if they worked.

- Ask about ice for your fingers, toes, and mouth.

- Ask about Claritin for Neulasta side effects.

- Be careful when you eat. Always have water with you.

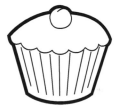

How can I look good while going through treatment?

Shopping!

Be honest with yourself, weren't you waiting for this moment? Weren't you waiting for the time when I tell you what I wore and how I handled how I looked? I read somewhere that the year of treatment for breast cancer ages how a woman looks more than anything else, and all I could think was, "NOT ME!" I was already 45, and I wasn't planning on speeding up the process.

I'll start at the top and share the decisions I faced and how I handled them.

I went bald. When your hair falls out, it hurts in a weird way. If you have ever gotten a kink in your hair, that is how it feels at first. I will say that being bald is liberating ... you get in the shower and wash top down and are out the door in minutes. I went most places without a hat or scarf; but sometimes I did need to cover my head, like at my kids' school where my oldest asked me not to show up bald.

I also bought two wigs. I first bought an expensive real hair wig that looked just like my hair. It was great until I let my wigmaker cut it. Big mistake! I should have taken it to my hairstylist who has cut my hair for 20 some-odd years and is a master with curls.

Unfortunately, after the wigmaker cut it, I looked like a reject from an 80s hair band. This wig was also difficult to put on as I had to use toupee tape to hold it onto my head. If I took it off, I had to use new tape to put it back on. Since I liked to take off my wigs, hats, etc. when I was in the car,

I had to plan for additional time to put my real-hair wig back on.

My other wig came from Godiva's wigs. It was cute, short, and straight. It looked great, but I didn't look like me when I wore it. This wig went on like a stocking cap, making it easy to take it off and put it back on in the car. However, I was almost arrested at school. No one recognized me as I was walking away with my daughter. I also couldn't cash a check at my bank because they didn't recognize me in the drive through until I took off my wig. DONE!

I also wore hats and scarves for sun protection and warmth. I bought hats at several places, but Nordstrom's hat selection was my favorite (and they have a great scarf selection, too). I only bought two hats before I went bald. I realized they would fit differently when I didn't have a full head of hair, so I decided to wait for more. With a newly bald head, soft hats are a must.

I went bald on Dec. 8, 2009. I needed something to sleep in because, although I am in Southern California, it gets below 30 degrees at night for five months of the year where I live. This also meant that driving the kids to school in the morning was COLD!

I bought something to sleep in off of a cancer site. Every time I rolled over in bed or moved my head, the hat would come down over my face like Dustin Hoffman's wig in *Tootsie* (did I just date myself?).

A friend of mine sent me a Buff® USA scarf and I loved it! These scarves are shaped like a tube and are soft, stretchy, and stay in place when you turn your head. They also come in fabrics with SPF, which is great because I didn't want my scalp to sunburn when I was outside.

An online scarf store called 4women.com carries BeauBeau® scarves. They offer tons of colors and patterns, pre-tied and stretchy so they go on like a hat (so easy and quick!). I had a couple of them.

I have friends who have worn wigs, and I know women who refused chemo because they didn't want to lose their hair. (Yep, they went against medical advice because of hair ... don't get me started.)

I don't know anything about the polar caps except that when I was going through my treatment, my doctor said they were seeing brain metastases in patients who used the old cold cap versions. That was all I needed to hear! There is a new version available, but I've never checked them out.

What to wear...

You'll want to be as warm and comfortable as possible when you go to chemo. Soft, comfy, and port-accessible clothing is ideal because the meds are cold, and the room is cold; you don't want to have to strip. I also iced my fingers and toes, so I wanted to be covered. My port was in my arm, so I always had a short sleeve or tank on under my other clothes. Pants that don't need a lot of work to remove are essential; I lived in yoga flare leggings and sweats. Because you will need to pee at some point while you are there, don't wear jeans with a button fly. You will be hooked up to an IV and learning to pole dance because your IV has to go with you, so you don't want to be fiddling with buttons or zippers! No jumpsuits no matter how fashionable they are right now. If you search "chemo clothes" online, you will find t-shirts with zippers to access your port. These are new so I didn't have them for my visits to the chemo chair.

If you are icing your toes, bring warm socks or Ugg boots to defrost your feet. I wore my cowboy boots the first time. I wanted to be cool and grounded in my cowboy boots at that first chemo. After that day, I wore Uggs. The idea of being able to sink my frozen feet into the warmth of soft fleece was dreamy, and the reality was even better. At the very least, if you are icing your feet, bring some warm socks for afterwards.

Comfy and warm clothes; layers are best

- Soft hats and scarves
- Pants you can take on and off with one hand
- Warm socks if you will be icing.

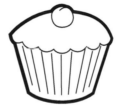

Side Effects

The Wonders of Modern Medicine Checklist

Ask your doctor about everything in this section. Everyone's cancer is different, and everyone's treatment is different. Things that were fine for me might not be for you.

My oncologist gave me seven pages of advice on what drug to use when. The office also had an on-staff nutritionist whom I saw once or twice.

I took prescription meds for nausea, which I highly recommend. I also had a prescription mouthwash for the mouth sores. I made use of some over-the-counter medications that they advised, such as Claritin. My doctor asked how bad my nausea had been when I was pregnant. I thought this was an interesting question, and I answered truthfully. They offer you the drugs for a multitude of reasons, which are particular to your type of chemo. The side effects differ according to which drugs you are on and your own personal constitution. I was told by another patient to not try to "get through" but to simply take what is prescribed as it is prescribed.

1. Write down what you do. I know I have said this before, but it makes things so easy. It is important to keep a careful record of what you took and if it worked, because I can almost guarantee that next time you won't remember. By the time you start chemo, your brain is overloaded with information, so write things down.

2. Utilize phone reminders. By putting your medication regimen on your phone, you'll be reminded when it's

time to take them. This way, if you have kids and are busy with them, you won't miss a dose.

3. Ask about homeopathic remedies. Ask your doctor before taking anything. I was able to use the one I asked about.

4. Ask about herbal meds. Ask your doctor before ingesting anything. I wasn't allowed to use these.

5. Consider taking glutamine. I was told to take this by the nutritionist at my oncologist's office. It is used to soothe the digestive track. It comes in a powder usually, and I put it in my morning smoothie. I might have mixed it into pudding – that seems like a good idea. Ask your doctor.

6. The trifecta—Neulasta, Claritin, and a heating pad. The Neulasta shot, which raises your white blood cell count to protective levels, can make you achy. My doctor recommended Claritin, so I took it. I also used a heating pad to soothe the aches, typically on day three. Ask your doctor.

7. Baking soda and salt for mouth sores. Ask your doctor, as your own personal health may prevent you from doing this; but you are not to swallow it—just gargle! At the suggestion of my oncologist, I rinsed my mouth with one-quarter teaspoon of each ingredient mixed in about two ounces of water six times a day. To help with this regimen, I mixed the baking soda and salt together in a container that I kept in my bathroom

along with small Dixie cups. Each morning, I would line up six Dixie cups and put approximately a quarter teaspoon of the mix into each cup. The amount isn't that important but the repetition is. Every time I went to the bathroom during the day, I would wash my hands, add warm water to one of the cups, and rinse my mouth and gargle with it. I also asked about and took powdered probiotics. I held them in my mouth for a bit before swallowing. I'm not sure if it helped, but it seemed like it would. Again, ask your doctor. For me, lining up the cups each day helped me to remember to rinse and gave me a visual as to how many times I had already done it. With kids, cooking, and recovering, I needed to have visual cues! I don't remember how long I rinsed my mouth, but it was probably for seven days. Ask your doctor!

8. Ask your doctor for nutrition advice. Many cancer centers have an on-staff nutritionist, which is really helpful. Some people can't have anything raw. For me, I had to increase my protein intake but was allowed raw vegetables and fruit. You don't want to interfere with the cancer medicine's work, so ask your doctor.

9. Check out hot sauce and Yale's cayenne taffy. I know some women who deal with mouth sores by eating cayenne saltwater taffy developed at Yale or by using Tabasco sauce. I think this has to do with increasing the pain to numb the pain. I am not sure, but I know some find it helpful. My stomach couldn't have dealt

with either one. I am enough of a lightweight regarding hot peppers without the addition of mouth sores!

10. Find a great moisturizer. My skin became very dry. To make matters worse, I went slamming into menopause, which made me more dry—everywhere. Coconut oil became my friend. You have to be careful when you use it as it can make the shower floor slippery. It also shouldn't go down your drain, as it will solidify, so make sure it ends up on your body. You can buy giant tubs of organic coconut oil at Costco. I used it everywhere. I also carried face cream with me to put on in the middle of the day. I used hand cream because I also washed my hands a lot. Washing just made the inherent dryness worse. I have my personal favorites and went for the heaviest and thickest I could find. I was dry before I had cancer. Thankfully, it has eased some in the past few years. I'm still dry, but I don't need to reapply in the middle of the day. I don't like chemicals in face and body products so I am a label reader. Luckily, the moisturizer I use in Colorado (really dry air there) fit the bill.

11. Take the drugs they give you. Ask about anything you might consider taking for side effects. Don't assume that if it's "natural" or "holistic" that it's good for you! Things are different when you're getting chemo.

12. One thing I remember about nausea is trying ginger—mostly in candied form. I also was told to try eating oranges or smelling oranges. It may sound weird but it seemed to help.

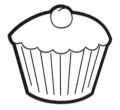

How do I deal
with sick friends
and relatives
(not to mention
perfect strangers)?

You would think this would be a no brainer, but some people just don't realize what they are doing. They will say things like, "Oh, I have a horrid cold, but I wanted to hug you anyway. I just had to see you." Really? You really had to see me? What part of compromised immune system do you not understand? Honestly, I had a friend who "had to" introduce me to her boyfriend—a doctor himself by the way—the week before chemo. He had a horrid cold and shook my hand. He then made sure to hug me before he left. My first chemo was delayed a week because of those "nice" gestures.

Remember the hand sanitizer I told you to buy? Put one in the front hall, on your bedside table, in each of your kid's lunchboxes and backpacks, on your desk, and in your cars. Wash your hands every time you get in the car. Ask visitors to wash their hands. This may seem like overkill, but it isn't. When I was in the chair for hydration after chemo number 1, there was a girl next to me who was waiting on her blood work. The results indicated that she was sick. She couldn't do chemo that day. It was going to be her first chemo. She was crushed. I couldn't imagine arriving at my first with all that apprehension and not being able to start! I thought, "I am NOT going to let that happen to me." I wanted my chemo treatments on time so I could finish before my birthday in March. You might think this would not be such a big deal, but I have had allergies my whole life, so I used to get every cold that walked by me. We were also supposed to have a horrible flu year that year,

41

so I was determined not to get sick. I was also aware that anything I got could be made worse by the lower immune system. Every time I got in the car, I would wash my hands, the steering wheel, and gearshift, especially after using the valet parking available at my cancer center. I would wash after paying with a credit card anywhere. I pushed elevator buttons with my knuckle or covered my hand with my sleeve. I even used my knee on one occasion.

Don't be afraid to send someone home, but be aware there could be consequences. I did this to one person, and she hasn't spoken to me since. It's been five years! She arrived with a sick child in tow, so I sent them home. I sent my daughter's friend home because she threw up at my house. Her parents thought it was because of the ride in the car. I wasn't taking any chances. I was due to have surgery in two days, so out the door they went. Her mom and I are still friends, as she understood. The ones that don't … well, you hope they never understand why this is important; because if they did understand, it would mean that they have someone in their lives with cancer. The bottom line is this: take care of yourself first. You're not being selfish, you are trying to stay alive.

If your kids are old enough, and mine were, they should know to go to Dad when they are sick. Make sure your kids understand that it's important you not contract anything that could delay your treatment.

- Wash your hands

- Use your knuckles or sleeve
- Send sick people home
- Stay away from sick people

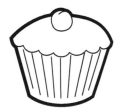

What do I eat?
Will I eat?

FOOD!

I will not tell you what to eat. That is for your doctor and nutritionist to do. I will tell you my experience.

I was fine and then ravenous. There was no moment of being a little hungry and looking for a snack. I went from zero to 60 instantly. My nutritionist said I needed to double my protein, so I carried nuts, nut bars, and peanut butter packs everywhere. The peanut butter packs were great; I enjoyed the ones with honey, too. I tried to eat healthy because that's what my body craved. Salads, omelets, and the like were my routine. I did a bit of fun eating in the beginning; I love dessert!

My weight went up about 15 to 20 pounds after my first chemo. I was dismayed, but at least I was able to eat. I had friends who couldn't, so I didn't complain. During my third chemo, I asked why they weighed me at every appointment. I learned that it was to make sure I was getting the right dose of chemo. I didn't want to add more chemo to my already serious load, so I paid more attention to eating healthy and was less ready to say yes to sweets after that. I stayed at the same weight after that, only fluctuating by a pound or two; still heavier than I would have liked, but no longer gaining.

Carry water with you, and don't eat without it. You need to stay hydrated. You may need to supplement with coconut water, Gatorade, etc. You may need to supplement lost vitamins and minerals, so ask the nutritionist. I needed more potassium and iron. I became anemic after my surgery and needed to rebuild my iron stores. I didn't take supplements; but I like steak and burgers, so I ate them with spinach. I really wasn't interested in liver so ... beef it was.

Sometimes it is about eating dessert first. Sometimes you need to treat yourself. One night I was at a party, and everything was too spicy as my mouth sores were active. So I could only eat dessert—honestly, that was the only thing I could eat!

- Carry a protein source
- Carry other snacks
- Carry water
- Ask about supplementation

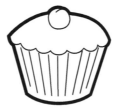

How do I find
faith, friends, and
moments to myself?

As moms, we put ourselves last all of the time. Now is the time to stop that. For the next few months in treatment, your life and your family's lives will revolve around how you feel, so make sure you do things that make you feel good. Find food you like, a God you trust, and friends that support you. Some people will disappear when you are sick. If they do, let them go. Some will drop everything to help. Find a way to connect with others via phone, Facebook, or a blog. The friends who support you are invaluable. Keep them close.

You must find the good and the positive in all of it. You must find the humor. I know it sounds impossible, but the whole situation is impossible, and you are working to fix that. Try to find a way to look on the bright side or at least don't dwell on the lousy. Your family needs you, and they need you to set an example of how to deal with this. I was very aware that I was teaching my kids how to deal with disappointment, fear, and frustration, so I showed them through my actions how to rise to the occasion. You need to do that, too. This doesn't mean you won't have tough times. And by all means, don't deny that things are hard, sad, frustrating, or scary. Just don't dwell on them. You are heading through a tunnel, so keep moving forward. There isn't anything to see to the right or the left, just straight ahead.

- Pray

- Meditate

- Live stream church services

- Keep in contact with friends through the phone, in person, Facebook, etc.

Should I troll the Internet – AKA – The Court of Public Opinion?

NO!

If you go looking for opinions, you will find them. They also won't always be positive or grounded in reality. If you ask your Facebook friend group for advice or opinions, I guarantee someone will tell you about how their aunt had that test or took that medication and then they found a brain tumor, and she died within the month. You don't need such things in your head. Hire a doctor you trust and go to it. Find an alternative doctor to work with, too, if that is something you want to do. Just know that everything should go through the oncologist first! Everything.

Some alternative, natural things work against chemo, so you don't want to add those to the mix. I had a friend ask about cleanses. I didn't want to cleanse; I wanted the cancer meds in me doing their work for as long as possible!

Stay away from negative people and situations. It is hard enough to stay positive in treatment; you don't need to add to the strain.

What does help is having a chemo sponsor, someone who has been through it. This person knows what it's like. They've walked your path. No matter how much someone loves you, they can't understand what you are going through unless they have been through it themselves. My doctor put me in touch with two women who were both moms, and then I found others. I also had an amazing group of nurses around me.

Helping someone else helps you, too. There is always some-one who has just received a diagnosis. You can help by talking to them or to the loved ones in the chairs near you.

- Don't troll the internet

- Find a friend who's been through it

- Help someone else

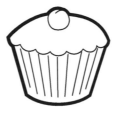

Will I feel like exercising?

Maybe. Maybe not.

My pattern was like this:

Day one: Chemo day, then rest at my mom's house afterwards

Day two: Go to center for hydration; pick up macaroons to take home

Day three: Feel pretty lousy. Able to walk to corner of our property and back a couple of times.

Day four: Walk to the corner and back a couple of times.

Day five: Walk the circle, which is a short quarter mile route.

Day six: Feel better; walking more.

I found that I needed to move my body and walking worked. It was winter, so I couldn't swim, and I don't know if I would have been allowed to anyway. Some people go to yoga class on chemo day. I felt too disconnected from my body to do that. The important thing is to do what feels good and what makes you happy. A walk on the beach, playing catch with your kid or dog, do whatever brings you joy and has you moving at least a little bit. The important thing is to do something that gets you up and out of bed. Believe me; there will be days when that is the last thing you feel like doing. Getting outside will do a lot for your point of view and your attitude.

- Walk
- Get outside
- Move your body

How do I volunteer at school?

Every school needs parent volunteers. My kids' school was no different. In May 2009, I was asked to teach Creative Writing to the sixth graders. It was a perfect job, and I jumped at the chance. I would also teach literature, the novel, as I asked to do that as well. I knew these two classes would inform each other and make it easy to use examples. I spent the summer planning and creating my courses and began teaching the second week of school. Then I was diagnosed. We figured out how I could teach over Skype. It didn't always work. One time, I threw my hands up in exasperation and jumped in my car to teach in the room … with the doors open and me standing in the doorway! I didn't take that risk again, but I loved teaching so much I had to make it work.

It may be hard, but choose not to be in the classroom. Bake cookies, drop things off, make phone calls, design the invitations to the events, but don't be in the classroom if you can help it. The way we get through chemo is to see and hold onto the date of the last chemo. Try your best to stay well, and don't risk the crowds. If you are dealing with metastatic disease, your life is different; and you will know when you are able to risk a crowd. For those of us with stage 0, 1, 2, or 3, we can plan for the end of chemo, and we need to. This was my experience. You may choose differently.

I chose just a few things to risk:

- My daughter's spelling bee with me in the back by the door in a mask

- That one day of teaching
- My friend's birthday party after chemo 3
- Seeing the Sherlock Holmes movie with Robert Downey, Jr., in a mask by the door
- Thanksgiving and Christmas Eve with my family, and
- My daughter's birthday dinner in December with two of her friends and my mom.

That was it. All were carefully planned events, and no one came near me who was sick. I made it through my treatment and reduced social exposure. It was, after all, only a four-and-one-half months' restriction. I just didn't need to be that social. If you work in an office, you have to mitigate exposure as much as possible. Meet outside, open your windows, get a tiny air purifier, if there is one, and break out the hand sanitizer.

- Volunteer by doing things outside of school. Donate, design, make phone calls, drop off supplies
- Only go to the really important things

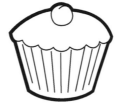

Why did I start
burning the
pancakes?

I have always talked to myself. It was great when I got a dog because I had someone to listen. Then when the kids came along, I had a captive audience that now never really wants to hear my stories.

With cell phone earpieces, I can walk down the street reciting my to-do list, and people think I am on the phone!

I can't remember if it was during or after chemo, but I started burning things. I couldn't multitask anymore. I had too many thoughts, too much chemo brain, and too many things that were overwhelming. I learned a new trick that saved our pancakes (and other things). When I turned away from the stove I would say, "The pancakes are on the stove." This would help me remember while I was cutting fruit or making a lunch. Now I had a really good reason to talk to myself!

As I have mentioned above, I wrote many things down, especially my medications and results. I used visual cues, as in the lining up of the Dixie cups to remind me to rinse my mouth. I put post-it notes on my mirror and reminders in my Smartphone. My great grandmother, who never had cancer, balanced so many things at once that she would write things down and pin them to her dress or shirt. Once she did something, she would remove the note. At the end of the day, she knew what was still left to accomplish.

The term "chemo brain" is a forgetfulness or fogginess that comes to some patients (me!). It was more prominent after I finished chemo, but that was also when I started to demand more of myself. Add chemo brain to instant menopause (me again!), and the mental fogginess is even more pronounced. The forgetfulness has improved over time. Some things ease and some issues you simply learn to accommodate.

- Write it down even if you never had to before

- Use a calendar and set reminders on your phone (I set them to remind me of things when I get home)

- Actually speak aloud what you are doing as you are doing it, whether you are burning the pancakes or anything else.

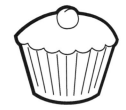

How did I
make decisions?

With a cancer diagnosis, making decisions becomes a full-time job. The decisions are always life and death even when they aren't.

I began having a hard time seeing all the ramifications of a question. "Mom, can I go to Jane's house on Saturday at 1:00?" I would say sure and then remember that we were supposed to be at a tennis lesson or something at 2:00 and have to say no later. I angered my family repeatedly, so I started by saying, "I have to think about it," which also bugged them. I would then check with the calendar and my husband to make sure we could do those things.

I also had a hard time making decisions. I think it was partly because I wasn't able to see the ramifications and also because so many decisions when you begin treatment are life and death. For decisions like what to remove, what treatment is best, what chemo should be done, whether radiation is necessary, etc., we patients and the doctors are gambling with odds and experiments. "This worked for this group with this type of cancer so it might work for you." It is one big question mark. If it wasn't, then everyone would survive and no one would experience a reoccurrence. To help with these decisions, making a pro/con list might help.

Sometimes it is best just to let your spouse make the decision. And then don't question it.

- Don't make decisions on the fly

- Check the calendar, with the spouse, with the child-care folks, etc.

- Make a list of pros and cons

- Let the spouse do it

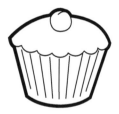

So there you have it.

Sixteen questions, a few checklists, and, hopefully, I have helped you plan your life for the next few months. Just remember to live in the moment. Hang out with your kids and husband. The girls and I used to go for muffins every Wednesday as they had a late start that day. On Mondays and Fridays we sat with a friend of ours on the couch and watched "Say Yes to the Dress." We lived in the midst. I went to soccer games and I went to bed early. I did their hair and I watched movies on demand with my husband. We went for walks. The lesson is not to stop living, but also rest and go to bed early. Visit my blog at angeliquelamour. com and head back to 2009 to see how I handled it. I promise it is a positive place to hang out. I was so tired of scary books and blogs that I was determined to write positively about my experience. I also hoped I would help others look at the positive side of things. Hang in there and stay where your feet are firmly planted—in the present.

Questions and Helpful Hints in a Nut Shell;
AKA Troubleshooting Guide

1: I Have Cancer; How Do I Tell My Kids?

- Keep it simple
- Answer the questions that are asked
- Don't make promises until you know you can make them come true

2: What Kind of Help Will I Need?

- Say yes to people who offer to help
- Get rides for chemo day for yourself and chemo day plus two more for your kids
- Let other parents know you won't need them to drive every day, and you will return the favor the week after
- Housekeeping help is terrific

3: What Should I Do Before Treatment Begins?

- A Checklist

4: What Can Spouses, Family Members, and Friends Do?

- Say yes
- Ask for help

5: Shall I Get a Port?

- Say yes to the port
- Frost a cupcake with the Lidocaine cream

6: What Will the Treatment and After Effects Be Like?

- Write it down: appointments, what drugs you take, and if they work
- Ask about ice for your fingers and toes, and mouth
- Ask about Claritin for Neulasta side effects
- Be careful when you eat. Always have water with you.

7: How Can I Look Good While Going Through Treatment?

- Comfy and warm clothes; layers are best
- Soft hats and scarves
- Pants you can take on and off with one hand
- Warm socks if you will be icing your toes

8: Side Effects and The Wonders of Modern Medicine

- A Checklist

9: How Do I Deal with Sick Friends and Relatives?

- Wash your hands
- Use your knuckles, sleeve or knee
- Send sick people home
- Stay away from sick people

10: What Do I Eat? Will I Eat?

- Carry a protein source
- Carry snacks
- Carry water
- Ask about supplementation

11: How Do I Find Faith, Friends, and Moments to Myself?

- Pray
- Meditate
- Live Stream Church Services
- Keep in Contact with Friends

12: Should I Troll the Internet aka: The Court of Public Opinion?

- Don't troll the Internet
- Find a friend who has been through it
- Help someone else

13: Will I Feel Like Exercising?

- Walk
- Get outside
- Move your body

14: How Do I Volunteer at School?

- Volunteer by doing things outside of school. Donate, design, make phone calls, drop off supplies
- Only go to the really important things

15: Why Did I Start Burning the Pancakes?

- Write it down even if you never had to before
- Use a calendar and set reminders on your phone (I set mine to remind me of things when I get home)
- Actually speak aloud what you are doing as you are doing it, whether you are burning the pancakes or anything else!

16: How Did I Make Decisions?

- Don't make decisions on the fly
- Check the calendar, with the spouse, with the child-care folks, etc.
- Make a list of pros and cons
- Let the spouse do it

Glossary

Some terms you don't know at the beginning but soon will!

BRCA I and II – These are genes that show up in certain families and populations that predict chances of breast and ovarian cancer. Not everyone carries them but some do, and it is important to know if you do so you can make decisions accordingly

Chemo – Taxotere and Carboplatin – Chemotherapy is a method of treating cancer with IV or pill form drugs. The two written above are the ones I was on and are only two of what are numerous drugs available to treat various cancers.

EOB – Explanation of Benefits – These come from your insurance company with frightening regularity when you are a cancer patient.

Glutamine – An amino acid which helps with inflammation and protects the gastrointestinal tract; some doctors suggest it for their patients

Herbal medicine – This is the use of a plant's seeds, berries, roots, leaves, bark, or flowers as medicine

Herceptin – A medicine used to treat HER2 positive cancer; for me this was an IV drug that I took every 21 days for a year with very few side effects (I felt dehydrated); not as tough in the side effect department as the other chemo drugs

Homeopathic medicine – Homeopathy is based on the idea that "like cures like." The idea is to use tiny amounts of a substance to cure a person (much like allergy immunizations or early inoculations but at a much smaller dose) There is a great deal online about this; and for me, I was allowed to use one such remedy.

Lidocaine – This is a numbing agent, and they may give this to you in a cream form to help numb the skin before they access your port for chemo.

Neulasta – A prescription medication used to help lower your chances of infection due to a low white blood cell count. I was given this the day after my chemo.

Port or Port-a-cath – This is a small, valve-type thing that is placed under the skin and has a catheter connected to it that leads to a vein. Usually these are placed in the upper chest or the arm, and you can receive chemo through it as well as have blood drawn from it. That way they only have to go through your skin once a visit. I had blood drawn and three chemo drugs and then hydration given the next day all through one access of my port.

Helpful Things

Buffusa.com – This is the place for the tube scarf that I slept in to keep my head warm. I also wore these when walking to keep my skin safe from the sun! Lots of colors and some with spf fabric, as well as some heavy winter weight ones.

BeauBeau scarves – Available on 4women.com, these go on like a hat but look like a scarf. No messing around with tying them and they come in all sorts of colors, patterns and fabrics.

Supersalve.com – The moisturizer I used in Colorado and then imported to California for my super dry chemo/menopausal skin for power repair. I still use it, and there is a version with spf I use during the day.

Coconut oil – You can get this anywhere. Even Costco.

About the Author

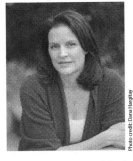

Photo credit: Dana Hargitay

Angelique L'Amour was born in Los Angeles, California. The daughter of author Louis L'Amour, she grew up in the household of a prolific writer where writing and storytelling were a way of life. In 1988 Angelique created and edited a volume of quotes from her father's works. Published by Bantam Doubleday Dell in 1988, *A Trail of Memories* spent 16 weeks on the *New York Times* bestseller list and was also a *Publisher's Weekly* bestseller for 1988.

Angelique has spent the past 20 years as a freelance editor working on academic papers, novels and film projects as well as writing content for two websites. She also created and taught a Creative Writing program for students from 8-80 and is contemplating developing that into an online and book course. Future projects include a spiritual self help book as well as several novels.

A wife, mother of two and a breast cancer survivor, time is also spent promoting early detection by teaching, speaking engagements and writing her blog, *My Story Right Now* which can be found through her website: angeliquelamour.com. Follow Angelique on Twitter, @LAmourAngelique or Facebook at www.facebook.com/angeliquelamourauthor.

About the Cover Artist

Denise Clemmensen has been an artist from the moment she could hold a crayon. Growing up in the San Fernando Valley, a suburb of Los Angeles she has been a graphic artist, a fine artist, a muralist, a children's singer-song-writer and a stay-at-home mom. Her illustrations can be seen in several educational books and a few e-books. Her first picture book "Just Because" written by Amber Housey won the Gelett Burgess Children's Book Award, a Mom's Choice Award and was picked by Creative Child as one of their 2012 Books of the year. Visit Denise at her website: deniseclemmensen.com

Praise for
A Trail of Memories,
The Quotations of Louis L'Amour

"It is a treasured keepsake of a wonderful friend and favorite American Writer. Thank you, Angelique, for sharing your work with us."

> — President Ronald Reagan

"It will delight them that she has captured so well by her selection the essence of the man as a gifted writer. Her introduction is of special interest as a testament to a most enviable family life with her father, mother and brother. In three pages it gives parents guidelines that merit the attention of professional counselors. *A Trail of Memories* holds a treasure for everyone on the trail of words to express what we feel and think and so seldom can or do say."

> — Evelyn Oppenheimer, *Dallas Times Herald*

Made in the USA
Middletown, DE
16 December 2019